MIND DIET COOKBOOK FOR SENIORS OVER 60

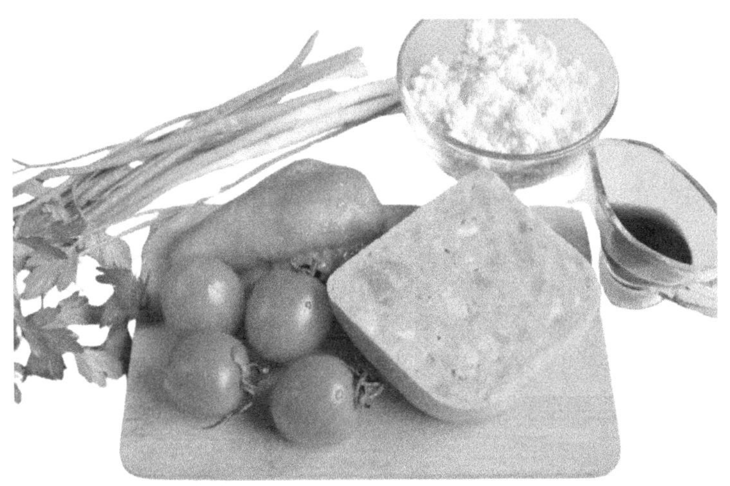

Enjoy meals designed to promote cognitive health and improve brain function.

Misty j. Font

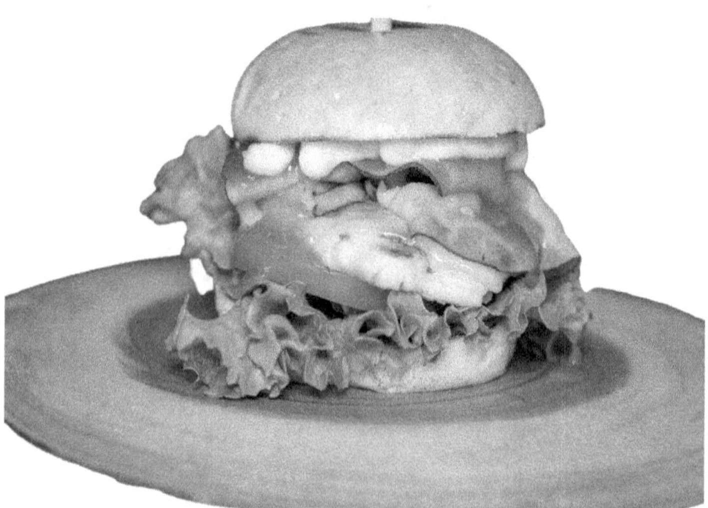

Table of Content

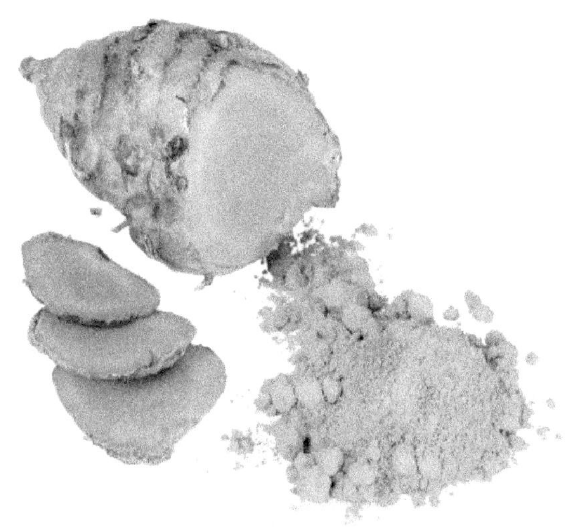

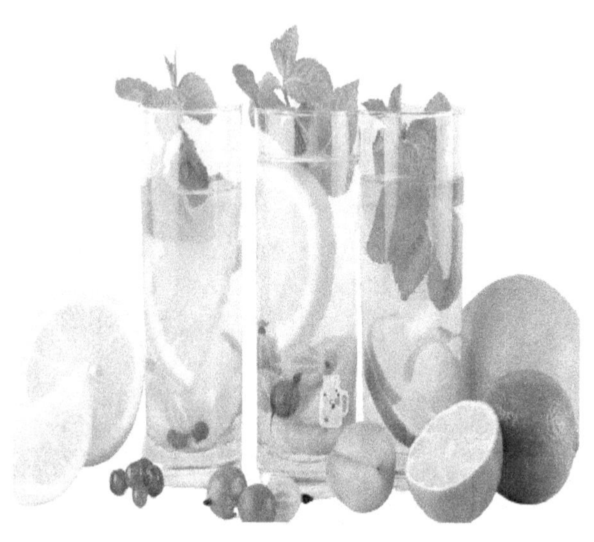

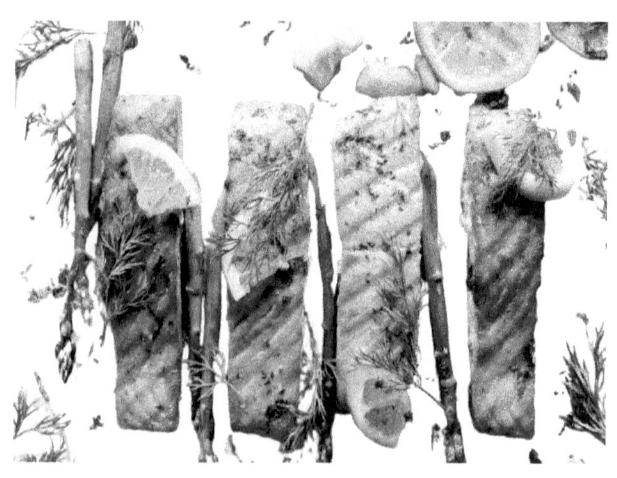

INTRODUCTION

Philip had always taken pride in his independence and vitality. At sixty-three, he enjoyed his daily walks through the park, his regular tennis games, and the satisfaction of preparing nutritious meals in his cozy kitchen. However, life had a way of throwing unexpected challenges at him, and Philip found himself dealing with a health issue that threatened to disrupt his active lifestyle.

It started with subtle signs—a brief moment of forgetfulness, a hint of fatigue that lasted longer than usual. Philip initially dismissed them, attributing them to normal wear and tear with age. But as the weeks passed, the signs became more pronounced, making him increasingly concerned about his health. A visit to his doctor confirmed his fears: Philip was experiencing early signs of cognitive decline, which required immediate attention and proactive measures to manage.

Determined not to let this setback define him, Philip began a journey of self-discovery and empowerment. He began researching ways to improve brain health and cognitive function in seniors. That's when he discovered the Mind Diet Cookbook, a comprehensive guide designed specifically for people over sixty, with a wealth of recipes to nourish both body and mind.

Philip eagerly embraced the cookbook's principles, fueled by a renewed sense of purpose. He stocked his kitchen with a variety of vibrant fruits, leafy greens, whole grains, and heart-healthy fats, which are the foundation of the Mind Diet. Gone were the days of processed foods and sugary snacks; instead, Philip found joy in experimenting with new ingredients and flavors, each dish carefully crafted to promote brain health.

As he immersed himself in the culinary journey ahead of him, Philip realized the transformative power of food as medicine. He marveled at how nutrient-dense foods not only fueled his body but also energized his mind, sharpening his focus and improving his clarity of thought. The foggy moments of confusion vanished, leaving behind a renewed sense of mental acuity and cognitive vitality.

The Mind Diet, however, provided benefits that extended far beyond cognitive health. Philip felt a profound sense of connection with each wholesome meal he prepared—to his body, to the earth, and to the simple joys of intentionally and mindfully nourishing oneself. Food was no longer viewed as mere sustenance; instead, Philip saw it as a form of self-care, a daily ritual with meaning and purpose.

As the weeks turned into months, Philip's commitment to the Mind Diet produced remarkable results. His cognitive function improved, his energy levels increased, and his enthusiasm for life returned. Gone were the fears of decline and dependency, and in their place stood a man empowered by the knowledge that he was in control of his own health and wellbeing.

Today, as Philip reflects on his recovery journey, he feels grateful and humble. He is aware that the road ahead may still be difficult, but armed with the knowledge of the Mind Diet Cookbook, he faces the future with confidence and resilience. For Philip, the journey to recovery has been more than just a quest for health; it has been a journey of self-discovery, a testament to the power of resilience, and a celebration of the limitless potential that we all possess.

Understanding The Mind Diet

The Mind Diet is more than just a fad; it is a scientifically supported approach to nutrition that has gained widespread attention for its profound impact on cognitive health. The Mind Diet, which is based on the Mediterranean and DASH (Dietary Approaches to Stop Hypertension) diets, focuses on eating nutrient-dense foods that promote brain health. The Mind Diet, which prioritizes whole grains, fruits, vegetables, nuts, and lean proteins while limiting processed foods, red meats, and saturated fats, is an effective tool for maintaining cognitive function and lowering the risk of age-related cognitive decline.

Benefits for Seniors over 60

The Mind Diet can have a transformative effect on seniors over the age of 60. As we age, maintaining cognitive vitality becomes increasingly important, and the Mind Diet provides a comprehensive approach to brain health. Seniors can nourish their brains, improve memory, sharpen focus, and lower their risk of neurodegenerative diseases such as Alzheimer's and dementia by eating nutrient-dense foods high in antioxidants, vitamins, and minerals. Furthermore, following the Mind Diet can improve overall physical well-being, such as heart health, weight management, and mood - all of which are important aspects of graceful aging.

How To Use This Cookbook

Navigating a new dietary regimen can be overwhelming, but don't worry - this cookbook is your guide to success. Here's how to make the best of it:

1.Explore Mindful Recipes: Dive into our collection of delicious and nutritious recipes designed to adhere to the Mind Diet's principles. From vibrant breakfast smoothies to filling dinner entrees and guilt-free desserts, there's something for every taste and occasion.

2. Embrace Variety: Variety is the spice of life—and the key to a well-balanced diet. Experiment with different ingredients, flavors, and cooking methods to keep your meals interesting and your taste buds satisfied.

3. Plan Ahead: Use our weekly meal planner and shopping tips to simplify your grocery shopping and meal preparation. By planning ahead of time, you can save time, reduce food waste, and increase your chances of success on your Mind Diet journey.

4. Practice Mindful Eating: Eating mindfully is an essential component of the Mind Diet philosophy. Take time to enjoy each bite, chew slowly, and pay attention to your body's hunger and fullness cues. By developing a stronger connection with your food, you will not only improve digestion but also gain a greater appreciation for the nourishment it provides.

5. Stay Informed: Knowledge equals power. Take advantage of the additional resources in this cookbook, such as recommended reading and online resources, to gain a better understanding of the Mind Diet and stay up to date on the latest developments in brain health and nutrition.

Chapter 1: Starting

Beginning the Mind Diet journey is an exciting step toward improving both physical and cognitive well-being. In Chapter 1, we lay the groundwork for your culinary adventure by delving into the Mind Diet's fundamentals and providing you with the tools and knowledge you'll need to succeed.

The Mind Diet Basics

What is The Mind Diet?

The Mind Diet is a lifestyle approach to eating that prioritizes foods high in nutrients known to promote brain health. The Mind Diet, based on the Mediterranean and DASH diets, emphasizes whole, minimally processed foods like fruits, vegetables, whole grains, nuts, legumes, and lean proteins. These nutrient-dense foods contain antioxidants, vitamins, and minerals that nourish the brain, reduce inflammation, and improve cognitive function.

Key Principles for Seniors

For seniors over the age of 60, adopting the Mind Diet can be transformative. The Mind Diet's key principles perfectly align with the nutritional needs of older adults, providing a delicious and sustainable way to support brain health as you age. Seniors can improve their overall health and vitality by eating a variety of colorful fruits and vegetables, incorporating heart-healthy fats from sources such as olive oil and nuts, and limiting red meat and processed foods.

Kitchen essentials

Essential Equipment

To begin your Mind Diet journey, you'll need a few basic kitchen tools to help you prepare delicious and nutritious meals with ease. From sharp knives and cutting boards to versatile cookware and small appliances, having the right tools on hand can make all the difference in your culinary adventures.

Pantry Staples

Stocking your pantry with essential ingredients is critical to success on the Mind Diet. Maintaining a well-stocked pantry ensures that you always have the ingredients for healthy and flavorful meals on hand. Whole grains, canned beans, olive oil, herbs and spices, and nuts and seeds are all versatile ingredients that can be used to make a variety of Mind Diet-friendly dishes.

Shopping Tip for Seniors

Navigating the grocery store can be difficult, especially for seniors. But don't worry; with these shopping tips, you'll be able to navigate the aisles with ease and confidence. Making and sticking to a list, shopping the perimeter of the store for fresh produce, and limiting processed foods are all strategies that will help you make healthy choices and stay on track with your Mind Diet goals.

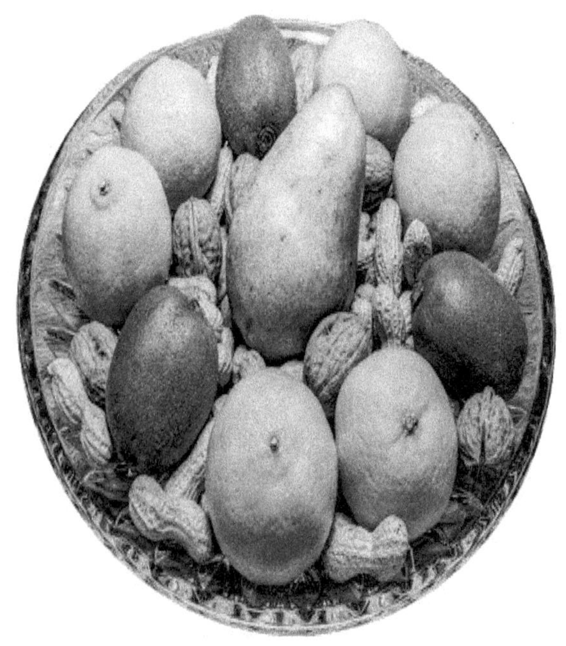

Chapter 2: Breakfast Recipes

Berry Blast Smoothie

Ingredients:

- 1 cup mixed berries (strawberries, blueberries, raspberries) -
- 1 handful spinach -
- 1/2 cup Greek yogurt
- One-half cup almond milk
- One tablespoon of honey (optional).

Instructions:

1. Combine all of the ingredients in a blender.
2. Blend until smooth and creamy.
3. Pour into a glass and drink immediately.

Avocado toast with poached egg

Ingredients:

- 1 slice whole grain bread, 1/2 ripe avocado.

- One egg - Salt and pepper to taste -

Instructions:

1. Toasted the bread until golden brown.

2. Mash the avocados and spread them on the toast.

3. Cook the egg to your preferred doneness and place it on top of the avocado.

4. Season with salt and pepper, then serve immediately.

Whole grain pancakes with blueberry compote

Ingredients:

- 1 cup whole wheat flour and 1 tablespoon baking powder.
- 1 tablespoon of honey or maple syrup.
- One cup almond milk.
- 1 egg

- 1 cup blueberries, fresh or frozen.

Instructions:

1. In a mixing bowl, combine the flour, baking powder, honey or maple syrup, almond milk, and egg. Whisk until smooth.
2. Place a nonstick skillet over medium heat and lightly coat with cooking spray.
3. Pour 1/4 cup batter into the skillet for each pancake.
4. Cook until bubbles appear on the surface, then flip and cook until golden brown on the opposite side.
5. In a small saucepan, cook the blueberries over medium heat until they begin to burst.
6. Serve the pancakes with warm blueberry compote on top.

Mediterranean omelette

Ingredients:

1. Two eggs.

2. 1/4 cup diced tomatoes,

3. 1/4 cup chopped spinach,

4. 2 tablespoons sliced olives,

5. 2 tablespoons crumbled feta cheese,

6. and 1 teaspoon olive oil.

7. Season with salt and pepper to taste.

Instructions:

1. In a mixing bowl, whisk together the eggs until thoroughly combined.

2. Heat olive oil in a nonstick skillet over medium heat.

3. Pour the eggs into the skillet, swirling to evenly coat the bottom.

4. Cook until the edges begin to set, then spread the tomatoes, spinach, olives, and feta cheese over one half of the omelette.

5. Fold the other half of the omelette over the filling and cook for an additional minute, or until the cheese melts.

6. Transfer the omelette to a plate, season with salt and pepper, and serve hot.

Overnight Oatmeal with Almond Butter

Ingredients:

- 1/2 cup rolled oats,
- 1/2 cup almond milk,
- and 1 tablespoon chia seeds.
- 1 tablespoon almond butter
- 1/2 sliced banana.
- One tablespoon of honey or maple syrup (optional)

Instructions:

1. In a mason jar or bowl, mix together the rolled oats, almond milk, chia seeds, and almond butter.

2. Mix well, then cover and refrigerate overnight.

3. Stir the oats in the morning, then top with sliced banana and a drizzle of honey or maple syrup, as desired.

4. Eat it cold or warm it in the microwave before serving.

Greek Yogurt Parfait With Granola and Berries

Ingredients:

- 1/2 cup Greek yogurt.
- Use 1/4 cup granola and
- 1/4 cup mixed berries (strawberries, blueberries, raspberries).
- One tablespoon of honey or maple syrup (optional)

Instructions:

1. In a glass or bowl, combine the Greek yogurt, granola, and mixed berries.

2. Layer the ingredients until they are all used up.

3. Optional: Drizzle with honey or maple syrup.

4. Serve immediately and savor the creamy, crunchy, sweet flavors.

Spinach and Mushroom Frittata

Ingredients:

- Four eggs.
- Add 1 cup chopped spinach and
- 1/2 cup sliced mushrooms.
- Add 1/4 cup diced onion and
- 1/4 cup shredded mozzarella cheese.
- One teaspoon olive oil.
- Season with salt and pepper to taste.

Instructions:

1. Preheat the oven to 350°F/175°C.

2. In a bowl, beat the eggs until well combined and season with salt and pepper.

3. Heat the olive oil in an oven-safe skillet over medium heat.

4. Sauté the onion and mushrooms until softened.

5. Cook the spinach until wilted.

6. Pour the beaten eggs into the skillet and distribute the vegetables evenly.

7. Add the shredded mozzarella cheese on top.

8. Place the skillet in the preheated oven for 15-20 minutes, or until the frittata has set and turned golden brown on top.

9. Cut into wedges and serve hot or room temperature.

Whole Wheat Banana Nut Muffins

Ingredients:

- 1 cup whole wheat flour and
- 1/2 teaspoon baking soda.

- One-half teaspoon baking powder
- 1/4 teaspoon of salt.
- two ripe bananas, mashed
- 1/4 cup honey or maple syrup.
- 1/4 cup unsweetened apple sauce
- 1/4 cup chopped walnuts.
- 1 egg
- 1/4 cup almond milk.

Instructions:

1. Preheat the oven to 350°F/175°C and line a muffin tin with paper liners.
2. In a bowl, combine the flour, baking soda, baking powder, and salt.
3. In a separate bowl, combine mashed bananas, honey or maple syrup, applesauce, chopped walnuts, egg, and almond milk.
4. Stir the wet ingredients into the dry ingredients until just combined.

5. Distribute the batter evenly between the muffin cups.

6. Bake for 18–20 minutes, or until a toothpick inserted in the center comes out clean.

7. Let cool in the muffin tin for 5 minutes, then transfer to a wire rack to cool completely.

Sweet Potato & Spinach Breakfast Hash

Ingredients:

- 1 medium peeled and diced sweet potato
- 1 cup baby spinach
- 1/4 cup diced onion
- 1/4 cup diced bell pepper
- 2 eggs
- One tablespoon of olive oil.
- Season with salt and pepper to taste.

Instructions:

1. Heat the olive oil in a skillet over medium heat.

2. Cook the sweet potato until tender and golden brown, about 8-10 minutes.

3. Cook the diced onions and bell pepper in the skillet until softened.

4. Add the baby spinach and cook until wilted.

5. Create two wells in the hash mixture and crack an egg into each.

6. Cover the skillet and cook for about 3-5 minutes, or until the eggs are firm to the touch.

7. Season with salt and pepper, then serve hot.

Quinoa Breakfast Bowl with Mixed Berries

Ingredients:

- 1/2 cup cooked quinoa,
- 1/4 cup mixed berries (strawberries, blueberries, raspberries), and
- 2 tablespoons chopped nuts (almonds,

- walnuts, pecans).

- 1 tablespoon of honey or maple syrup.

- One-quarter teaspoon cinnamon

- 1/4 cup Greek yogurt.

Instructions:

1. In a bowl, combine the cooked quinoa, mixed berries, chopped nuts, honey or maple syrup, and cinnamon.

2. Optionally, top with Greek yogurt and additional berries.

3. Enjoy this protein-packed and fiber-rich breakfast bowl, warm or cold.

Egg and Vegetable Breakfast Muffins

Ingredients:

- 6 eggs.

- 1/2 cup diced bell pepper

- 1/2 cup diced zucchini

- 1/4 cup diced onion

- 1/4 cup chopped spinach

- 1/4 cup shredded cheese (either cheddar or mozzarella)

- Season with salt and pepper to taste.

Instructions:

1. Heat the oven to 350°F (175°C) and grease a muffin tin.

2. In a bowl, beat the eggs until well combined and season with salt and pepper.

3. Arrange the diced vegetables evenly in the muffin cups.

4. Pour the beaten eggs over the vegetables, filling each muffin cup approximately 3/4 full.

5. Sprinkle shredded cheese on top of each muffin.

6. Bake the muffins for 20-25 minutes, or until set and golden brown on top.

7. Allow to cool slightly before removing from the muffin tin.

8. Enjoy these protein-packed and portable breakfast muffins warm or at room temperature.

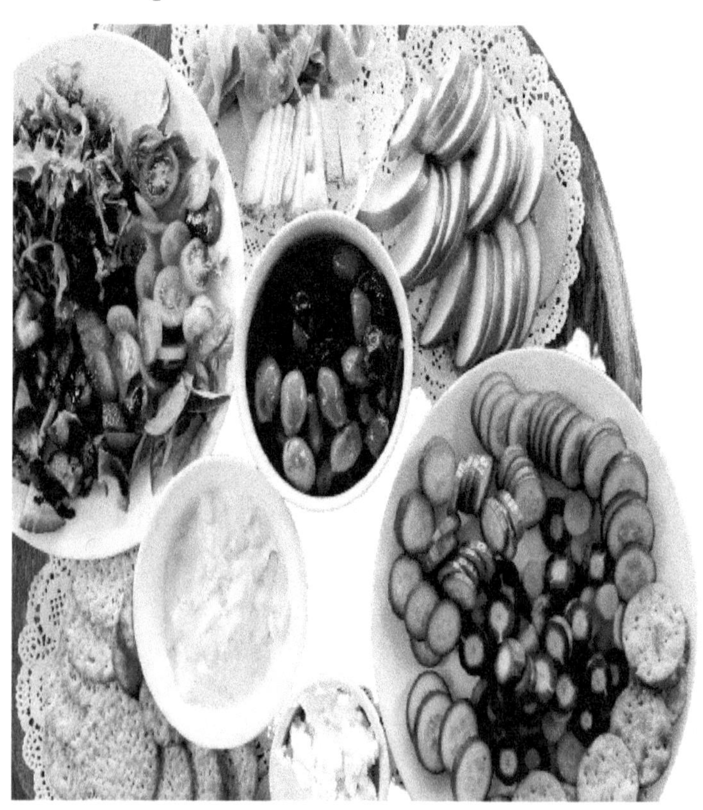

Chapter 3: Lunch recipes

Grilled salmon with lemon-dill sauce

Ingredients:

- 1 salmon fillet,

- 1 tablespoon olive oil.

- Season with salt and pepper to taste.

- Add 1/2 lemon juice.

- Use 1 tablespoon chopped fresh dill.

Instructions:

1. Preheat the grill to medium-high heat.

2. Coat the salmon fillet with olive oil and season with salt and pepper.

3. Grill the salmon for 4-5 minutes on each side, or until cooked through.

4. In a small bowl, combine the lemon juice and chopped dill.

5. Drizzle lemon-dill sauce over the grilled salmon before serving.

Turkey and Vegetable Stir Fry

Ingredients:

- 1 tablespoon olive oil
- 1 pound lean ground turkey
- 2 cups mixed vegetables (bell peppers, broccoli, carrots, snap peas)
- 2 minced garlic cloves.
- Two tablespoons of low-sodium soy sauce
- One teaspoon of sesame oil.
- Cooked brown rice to serve.

Instructions:

1. Heat the olive oil in a large skillet or wok over medium-high heat.
2. Cook the ground turkey until browned, breaking it up with a spoon.

3. Add the mixed vegetables and garlic to the skillet and cook until tender and crisp.

4. Add soy sauce and sesame oil, and cook for another 2-3 minutes.

5. Serve the turkey and vegetable stir-fry over cooked brown rice.

Quinoa-stuffed bell peppers

Ingredients:

- 4 large bell peppers,
- halved and seeded
- 1 cup cooked quinoa
- 1 cup black beans, drained and rinsed
- One cup of diced tomatoes
- 1/2 cup corn kernels
- 1/4 cup chopped fresh cilantro.
- Add 1 teaspoon cumin and 1/2 teaspoon chili powder.
- Season with salt and pepper to taste.

Instructions:

1. Preheat the oven to 375°F (190° C).

2. In a large bowl, combine the cooked quinoa, black beans, diced tomatoes, corn kernels, cilantro, cumin, chili powder, salt, and pepper.

3. Spoon the quinoa mixture into the halved bell peppers.

4. Arrange the stuffed bell peppers in a baking dish and cover with foil.

5. Bake for 25–30 minutes, or until the peppers are tender.

6. Serve the quinoa-stuffed bell peppers hot.

Lentil and Vegetable Soup

Ingredients:

- 1 tablespoon olive oil,
- 1 diced onion,
- 2 diced carrots, and
- 2 diced celery stalks.

- 2 garlic cloves, minced

- One cup dried lentils, rinsed and drained

- 4 cups of low-sodium vegetable broth,

- 1 bay leaf, and 1 teaspoon dried thyme.

- Season with salt and pepper to taste.

Instructions:

1. Heat the olive oil in a large pot over medium heat.

2. Cook the diced onion, carrots, and celery until softened.

3. Stir in the minced garlic and cook for an additional minute.

4. Place the dried lentils, vegetable broth, bay leaf, dried thyme, salt, and pepper in the pot.

5. Bring the soup to a boil, then reduce the heat and simmer for 20-25 minutes, or until the lentils are tender.

6. Remove the bay leaf before serving.

Chicken and vegetable skewers

Ingredients:

- 1 pound chicken breast, cut into chunks.
- Cut two bell peppers into chunks
- 1 sliced zucchini
- 1 chopped onion
- Eight wooden skewers soaked in water
- Add 2 tablespoons olive oil and 1 teaspoon garlic powder.
- one teaspoon dried oregano.
- Season with salt and pepper to taste.

Instructions:

1. Preheat the grill or grill pan on medium-high heat.
2. Thread chicken breast, bell peppers, zucchini, and onion onto skewers, alternating between them.

3. In a small bowl, combine the olive oil, garlic powder, dried oregano, salt, and pepper.

4. Brush the skewers with the olive oil mixture.

5. Grill the skewers for 8-10 minutes, turning occasionally, until the chicken is fully cooked and the vegetables are tender.

6. Serve the chicken and vegetable skewers hot from the grill.

Mediterranean Chickpea Salad

Ingredients:

- 1 can (15 ounces) drained and rinsed chickpeas
- 1 diced cucumber
- 1 cup cherry tomatoes (halved)
- 1/4 cup diced red onion
- Add 1/4 cup chopped fresh parsley,
- 1/4 cup crumbled feta cheese, and 2 tablespoons lemon juice.

- Add 2 tablespoons olive oil and 1 teaspoon dried oregano.
- Add salt and pepper to taste.

Instructions:

1. In a large mixing bowl, combine chickpeas, cucumber, cherry tomatoes, red onion, parsley, and feta cheese.
2. In a small bowl, combine the lemon juice, olive oil, dried oregano, salt, and pepper.
3. Pour dressing over chickpea mixture and toss to coat.
4. Serve the Mediterranean chickpea salad chilled or at room temperature.

Tuna Salad Lettuce Wraps

Ingredients:

- 1 can (5 ounces) drained tuna.
- Combine 1/4 cup diced celery,
- 1/4 cup diced red bell pepper,

- 2 tablespoons diced red onion, and 2 tablespoons Greek yogurt.
- One tablespoon of lemon juice.
- One teaspoon Dijon mustard.
- Season with salt and pepper to taste. - Butter the lettuce leaves.

Instructions:

1. In a bowl, mix together the tuna, celery, red bell pepper, red onion, Greek yogurt, lemon juice, Dijon mustard, salt, and pepper.
2. Mix until thoroughly combined.
3. Spoon the tuna salad onto the butter lettuce leaves.
4. Roll lettuce leaves to make wraps.
5. Serve tuna salad lettuce wraps chilled or room temperature.

Vegetable Frittata With Feta Cheese

Ingredients:

- 6 eggs.
- Add 1/4 cup milk, 1 tablespoon olive oil, 1/2 cup diced bell pepper,
- 1/2 cup diced zucchini,
- 1/4 cup diced onion, and
- 1/4 cup crumbled feta cheese.
- Add salt and pepper to taste

Brown rice and black bean burrito bowl

Ingredients:

- 1 cup cooked brown rice
- 1 cup black beans (drained and rinsed).
- 1/2 cup diced tomatoes.
- Add 1/4 cup diced red onion and 1/4 cup diced avocado.
- Two tablespoons of chopped cilantro
- Juice from 1/2 lime.
- Season with salt and pepper to taste.

Instructions:

1. In a bowl, combine cooked brown rice, black beans, tomatoes, red onion, avocado, and cilantro.

2. Drizzle the lime juice over the mixture and season with salt and pepper.

3. Stir until thoroughly combined.

4. Serve the brown rice and black bean burrito bowl immediately.

Caprese Salad With Balsamic Glaze

Ingredients:

- Two sliced ripe tomatoes.

- 4 oz fresh mozzarella cheese, sliced

- Use 1/4 cup fresh basil leaves and 2 tablespoons balsamic glaze.

- Season with salt and pepper to taste.

Instructions:

1. Arrange tomato and mozzarella slices on a serving platter, alternating them.

2. Place fresh basil leaves between tomato and mozzarella slices.

3. Drizzle balsamic glaze over salad.

4. Season with salt and pepper.

5. Serve immediately for a refreshing and light lunch option.

Spinach and Mushroom Quiche

Ingredients:

- One pre-made whole wheat pie crust - Four eggs.
- Chop 1 cup baby spinach.
- Slice 1 cup mushrooms.
- 1/2 cup shredded Swiss cheese.
- Half cup milk or unsweetened almond milk
- Season with salt and pepper to taste.

Instructions:

1. Preheat the oven to 375°F (190° C).

2. Place the pie crust into a pie dish and set aside.

3. In a skillet, cook the chopped spinach and sliced mushrooms until softened.

4. In a bowl, combine the eggs, shredded Swiss cheese, milk, salt, and pepper.

5. Stir in the sautéed spinach and mushrooms.

6. Pour the egg mixture into the pie crust.

7. Bake for 30-35 minutes, or until the quiche has set and the crust is golden brown.

8. Allow to cool slightly before slicing and serving.

Roasted Vegetables and Hummus Wrap

- *Ingredients:*
- 1 whole wheat tortilla,
- 2 tablespoons hummus,
- 1/2 cup roasted vegetables (bell peppers, zucchini, eggplant, onions),

- 1/4 cup baby spinach leaves, and 1 tablespoon crumbled feta cheese.

Instructions:

1. Spread the hummus evenly on the whole wheat tortilla.
2. Spread roasted vegetables, baby spinach leaves, and crumbled feta cheese on top of the hummus.
3. Roll the tortilla tightly to make a wrap.
4. If desired, cut in half and serve immediately.

shrimp and avocado salad

Ingredients:

- 8 ounces cooked shrimp, peeled and deveined
- 1 diced avocado
- 1 cup cherry tomatoes, halved.
- 1/4 cup diced red onion.
- Two tablespoons of chopped fresh cilantro
- 1 lime juice and 1 tablespoon olive oil.

- Season with salt and pepper to taste.

Instructions:

1. In a large mixing bowl, combine cooked shrimp, diced avocado, cherry tomatoes, diced red onion, and fresh cilantro.

2. Drizzle lime juice and olive oil over the salad.

3. Season with salt and pepper.

4. Gently toss the ingredients until evenly coated.

5. Serve the shrimp and avocado salad chilled or room temperature.

Whole wheat pasta primavera

Ingredients:

- 8 ounces whole wheat pasta, 1 tablespoon olive oil, and 2 minced garlic cloves.

- 1 cup mixed vegetables (e.g., bell peppers, broccoli, carrots, snap peas)

- 1/4 cup cherry tomatoes (halved)
- 1/4 cup grated parmesan cheese.
- Add salt and pepper to taste.

Instructions:

1. Cook whole wheat pasta according to the package instructions.
2. In a skillet, heat the olive oil over medium heat.
3. Add the minced garlic and cook until fragrant.
4. Add the mixed vegetables and cherry tomatoes to the skillet.
5. Cook until the vegetables are tender and crisp.
6. Mix cooked pasta into the vegetable mixture.
7. Sprinkle grated Parmesan cheese over the pasta.
8. Season with salt and pepper.
9. Serve the whole wheat pasta primavera hot.

Cauliflower Crust Pizza with Vegetables

Ingredients:

- 1 grated head of cauliflower - 1 egg
- 1/4 cup grated parmesan cheese.
- 1/2 teaspoon of dried oregano.
- One-half teaspoon garlic powder
- Add salt and pepper to taste.
- Use 1/4 cup pizza sauce.
- 1/2 cup shredded mozzarella cheese.
- 1/2 cup of mixed vegetables (bell peppers, mushrooms, onions).

Instructions:

1. Preheat the oven to 425°F (220°C).
2. In a mixing bowl, combine grated cauliflower, egg, Parmesan cheese, dried oregano, garlic powder, salt, and pepper.
3. Mix until thoroughly combined.

4. Shape the cauliflower mixture into a round crust on a parchment-lined baking sheet.

5. Bake the cauliflower crust for 15-20 minutes, until golden brown and set.

6. Spread the pizza sauce on the baked crust.

7. Sprinkle with shredded mozzarella and mixed vegetables.

8. Return the pizza to the oven and cook for another 10-12 minutes, or until the cheese is melted and bubbly.

9. Slice and serve the cauliflower crust pizza hot.

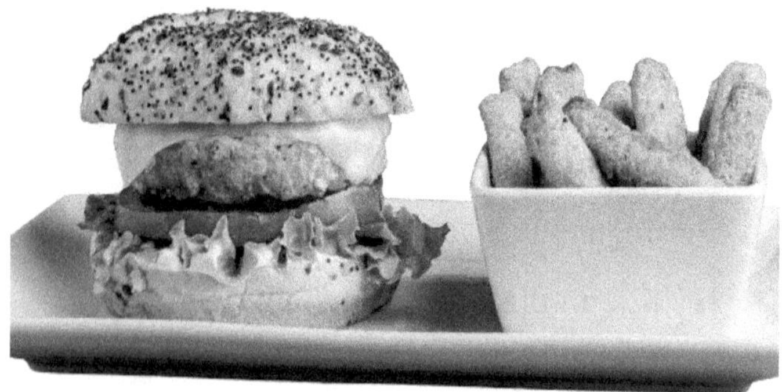

Chapter 4: Dinner Entrees

Baked Lemon Herb Chicken

Ingredients:

- 4 boneless, skinless chicken breasts,
- 2 tablespoons olive oil, and
- 2 minced garlic cloves.
- Zest and juice from 1 lemon
- Use 1 teaspoon dried thyme and 1 teaspoon dried rosemary.
- Season with salt and pepper to taste.

Instructions:

1. Preheat your oven to 375°F (190°C).
2. Arrange chicken breasts in a baking dish.
3. In a small mixing bowl, combine olive oil, minced garlic, lemon zest, lemon juice, dried thyme, rosemary, salt, and pepper.

4. Pour the marinade over the chicken breasts and coat them evenly.

5. Bake for 25-30 minutes, or until the chicken is tender and the juices run clear.

6. Serve hot, topped with fresh herbs if desired.

Salmon and asparagus foil packs

Ingredients:

- 4 salmon fillets
- 1 bunch of trimmed asparagus
- 2 tablespoons olive oil and
- 2 minced garlic cloves.
- Juice from 1 lemon
- Season with salt and pepper to taste.

Instructions:

1. Preheat your oven to 400°F (200°C).

2. Place each salmon fillet on a piece of aluminum foil that is large enough to fold over and seal.

3. Arrange asparagus around the salmon fillets.

4. In a small bowl, combine the olive oil, minced garlic, lemon juice, salt, and pepper.

5. Drizzle the olive oil mixture over the asparagus and salmon.

6. Fold the foil over the salmon and asparagus, forming a packet and sealing the edges tightly.

7. Place the foil packets on a baking sheet and bake for 15-20 minutes, or until the salmon and asparagus are tender.

8. Gently open the foil packets and serve hot.

Quinoa-stuffed bell peppers

Ingredients:

- 4 large bell peppers,
- halved and seeded
- 1 cup cooked quinoa
- 1 cup black beans,
- drained and rinsed

- One cup of diced tomatoes
- 1/2 cup corn kernels
- 1/4 cup chopped fresh cilantro.
- Add 1 teaspoon cumin and
- 1/2 teaspoon chili powder.
- Season with salt and pepper to taste.

Instructions:

1. Preheat your oven to 375°F (190°C).
2. In a large bowl, combine the cooked quinoa, black beans, diced tomatoes, corn kernels, cilantro, cumin, chili powder, salt, and pepper.
3. Spoon the quinoa mixture into the halved bell peppers.
4. Arrange the stuffed bell peppers in a baking dish and cover with foil.
5. Bake for 25–30 minutes, or until the peppers are tender.
6. Serve the quinoa-stuffed bell peppers hot.

Lentil and Vegetable Soup

Ingredients:

- 1 tablespoon olive oil,
- 1 diced onion,
- 2 diced carrots, and
- 2 diced celery stalks.
- garlic cloves, minced
- One cup dried lentils,
- rinsed and drained
- 4 cups of low-sodium vegetable broth,
- 1 bay leaf, and 1 teaspoon dried thyme.
- Season with salt and pepper to taste.

Instructions:

1. Heat the olive oil in a large pot over medium heat.
2. Cook the diced onion, carrots, and celery until softened.

3. Stir in the minced garlic and cook for an additional minute.

4. Place the dried lentils, vegetable broth, bay leaf, dried thyme, salt, and pepper in the pot.

5. Bring the soup to a boil, then reduce the heat and simmer for 20-25 minutes, or until the lentils are tender.

6. Remove the bay leaf before serving.

Chicken and Vegetable Stir-Fry

Ingredients:

- 1 tablespoon olive oil.
- Cut 1 pound of boneless,
- skinless chicken breasts into strips.
- 2 cups mixed vegetables (e.g., bell peppers, broccoli, carrots, snap peas) and 2 minced garlic cloves.
- Two tablespoons of low-sodium soy sauce
- One teaspoon of sesame oil.
- Cooked brown rice to serve.

Instructions:

1. Heat the olive oil in a large skillet or wok over medium-high heat.

2. Cook chicken strips until browned and cooked through.

3. Remove the chicken from the skillet and set it aside.

4. Place the mixed vegetables in the skillet and cook until tender-crisp.

5. Return the cooked chicken to the skillet and add the minced garlic.

6. Add the low-sodium soy sauce and sesame oil, and cook for another 2-3 minutes.

7. Serve the chicken and vegetable stir-fry over cooked brown rice.

Mediterranean Chickpea Salad

Ingredients:

- 1 can (15 ounces) drained and

- rinsed chickpeas

- 1 diced cucumber

- 1 cup cherry tomatoes (halved)

- 1/4 cup diced red onion

- Add 1/4 cup chopped fresh parsley,

- 1/4 cup crumbled feta cheese,

- and 2 tablespoons lemon juice.

- Add 2 tablespoons olive oil and

- 1 teaspoon dried oregano.

- Add salt and pepper to taste.

Instructions:

1. In a large mixing bowl, combine chickpeas, cucumber, cherry tomatoes, red onion, parsley, and feta cheese.

2. In a small bowl, combine the lemon juice, olive oil, dried oregano, salt, and pepper.

3. Pour dressing over chickpea mixture and toss to coat.

4. Serve the Mediterranean chickpea salad chilled or at room temperature.

Tuna Salad Lettuce Wraps

Ingredients:

- 2 cans (5 ounces each) of drained tuna.

- Combine 1/4 cup diced celery,

- 1/4 cup diced red bell pepper,

- 2 tablespoons diced red onion, and

- 2 tablespoons Greek yogurt.

- One tablespoon of lemon juice.

- One teaspoon Dijon mustard.

- Season with salt and pepper to taste. - Butter the lettuce leaves.

Instructions:

- In a bowl, mix together the tuna, celery, red bell pepper, red onion, Greek yogurt, lemon juice, Dijon mustard, salt, and pepper.

- Mix until thoroughly combined.

- Spoon the tuna salad onto the butter lettuce leaves.

- Roll lettuce leaves to make wraps.

- Serve tuna salad in lettuce.

Vegetable Frittata With Feta Cheese

Ingredients:

- 6 eggs.

- Add 1/4 cup milk,

- 1 tablespoon olive oil,

- 1/2 cup diced bell pepper,1/2 cup diced zucchini,

- 1/4 cup diced onion, and

- 1/4 cup crumbled feta cheese.

- Season with salt and pepper to taste.

Instructions:

1. Preheat the oven to 350°F/175°C.

2. In a bowl, combine the eggs, milk, salt, and pepper.

3. Heat the olive oil in an oven-safe skillet over medium heat.

4. Cook the diced bell pepper, zucchini, and onion in the skillet until softened.

5. Pour the egg mixture into the skillet and gently stir to distribute the vegetables evenly.

6. Sprinkle crumbled feta cheese on top.

7. Place the skillet in the preheated oven for 15-20 minutes, or until the frittata has set and the edges are golden brown.

8. Cut into wedges and serve hot.

Brown rice and black bean burrito bowl

Ingredients:

- 1 cup cooked brown rice
- 1 cup black beans (drained and rinsed).
- 1/2 cup diced tomatoes.
- Add 1/4 cup diced red onion and
- 1/4 cup diced avocado.
- Two tablespoons of chopped cilantro

- Juice from 1/2 lime.

- Season with salt and pepper to taste.

Instructions:

1. In a mixing bowl, combine the cooked brown rice, black beans, diced tomatoes, red onion, avocado, cilantro, lime juice, salt, and pepper.
2. Toss until thoroughly combined.
3. Serve the brown rice and black bean burrito bowl immediately.

Caprese Salad With Balsamic Glaze

Ingredients:

- Two sliced ripe tomatoes.

- 4 oz fresh mozzarella cheese,

- sliced

- Use 1/4 cup fresh basil leaves and 2 tablespoons balsamic glaze.

- Season with salt and pepper to taste.

Instructions:

1. Arrange tomato and mozzarella slices on a serving platter, alternating them.

2. Place fresh basil leaves between tomato and mozzarella slices.

3. Drizzle balsamic glaze over salad.

4. Season with salt and pepper.

5. Serve immediately for a refreshing and light dinner option.

Spinach and Mushroom Quiche

Ingredients:

- One pre-made whole wheat pie crust - Four eggs.
- Chop 1 cup baby spinach.
- Slice 1 cup mushrooms.
- 1/2 cup shredded Swiss cheese.
- Half cup milk or unsweetened almond milk
- Season with salt and pepper to taste.

Instructions:

1. Preheat your oven to 375°F (190°C).

2. Transfer the pie crust to a pie dish and set aside.

3. In a skillet, cook the chopped spinach and sliced mushrooms until softened.

4. In a bowl, combine the eggs, shredded Swiss cheese, milk, salt, and pepper.

5. Add the sautéed spinach and mushrooms.

6. Transfer the egg mixture to the pie crust.

7. Bake for 30-35 minutes, or until the quiche has set and the crust is golden brown.

8. Allow to cool slightly before slicing and serving.

Roasted Vegetables and Hummus Wrap

Ingredients:

*   1 whole wheat tortilla,

- 2 tablespoons hummus,

- 1/2 cup roasted vegetables (bell peppers, zucchini, eggplant, onions),

- 1/4 cup baby spinach leaves, and 1 tablespoon crumbled feta cheese.

Instructions:

1. Spread the hummus evenly on the whole wheat tortilla.

2. Spread roasted vegetables, baby spinach leaves, and crumbled feta cheese on top of the hummus.

3. Roll the tortilla tightly to make a wrap.

4. If desired, cut in half and serve immediately.

shrimp and avocado salad

Ingredients:

- 8 ounces cooked shrimp,

- peeled and deveined

- 1 diced avocado - 1 cup cherry tomatoes, halved.
- 1/4 cup diced red onion.
- Two tablespoons of chopped fresh cilantro
- 1 lime juice and 1 tablespoon olive oil.
- Season with salt and pepper to taste.

Instructions:

1. In a large mixing bowl, combine cooked shrimp, diced avocado, cherry tomatoes, diced red onion, and fresh cilantro.
2. Drizzle lime juice and olive oil over the salad.
3. Season with salt and pepper.
4. Gently toss the ingredients until evenly coated.
5. Serve the shrimp and avocado salad chilled or room temperature.

Whole wheat pasta primavera

Ingredients:

- 8 ounces whole wheat pasta,
- 1 tablespoon olive oil, and
- 2 minced garlic cloves.
- 1 cup mixed vegetables (e.g., bell peppers, broccoli, carrots, snap peas) -
- 1/4 cup cherry tomatoes (halved)
- 1/4 cup grated parmesan cheese.
- Add salt and pepper to taste.

Instructions:

1. Cook whole wheat pasta according to the package instructions.
2. In a skillet, heat the olive oil over medium heat.
3. Add the minced garlic and cook until fragrant.

4. Add the mixed vegetables and cherry tomatoes to the skillet.

5. Cook until the vegetables are tender and crisp.

6. Mix cooked pasta into the vegetable mixture.

7. Sprinkle grated Parmesan cheese over the pasta.

8. Season with salt and pepper.

9. Serve the whole wheat pasta primavera hot.

Cauliflower Crust Pizza with Vegetables

Ingredients:

- 1 grated head of cauliflower
- 1 egg
- 1/4 cup grated parmesan cheese.
- 1/2 teaspoon of dried oregano.
- One-half teaspoon garlic powder
- Add salt and pepper to taste. - Use 1/4 cup pizza sauce.
- 1/2 cup shredded mozzarella cheese.

- 1/2 cup of mixed vegetables (bell peppers, mushrooms, onions).

Instructions:

1. Pre-heat the oven to 425°F (220°C).

2. In a mixing bowl, combine grated cauliflower, egg, Parmesan cheese, dried oregano, garlic powder, salt, and pepper.

3. Mix until thoroughly combined.

4. Spread the cauliflower mixture.

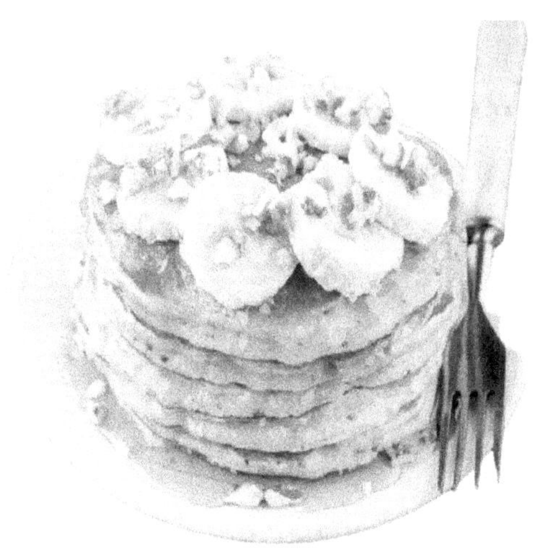

Chapter 5: Sides and Salads

Steamed Broccoli and Lemon

Ingredients:

- 2 cups broccoli florets and
- 1 tablespoon olive oil.
- Juice from 1/2 lemon.
- Season with salt and pepper to taste.

Instructions:

1. Steam broccoli florets until tender, about 5-7 minutes.
2. Drizzle with olive oil and lemon juice.
3. Sprinkle with salt and pepper before serving.

Quinoa Salad with Mixed Vegetables

Ingredients:

- 1 cup cooked quinoa,

- 1 cup mixed vegetables (bell peppers, cucumbers, cherry tomatoes),
- 2 tablespoons chopped fresh parsley,
- 2 tablespoons olive oil, and
- 1 tablespoon lemon juice.
- Season with salt and pepper to taste.

Instructions:

1. In a large bowl, combine cooked quinoa, mixed vegetables, and chopped parsley.
2. Drizzle with olive oil and lemon juice.
3. Season with salt and pepper.
4. Before serving, toss the ingredients until thoroughly combined.

Roasted Sweet Potatoes

Ingredients:

- 12 medium peeled and diced sweet potatoes
- 1 tablespoon olive oil
- 1 teaspoon smoked paprika.

- One-half teaspoon garlic powder

- Season with salt and pepper to taste.

Instructions:

1. Preheat your oven to 400°F (200°C).

2. Toss diced sweet potatoes in a bowl with olive oil, smoked paprika, garlic powder, salt, and pepper to coat evenly.

3. Arrange the sweet potatoes in a single layer on a baking sheet.

4. Roast in a preheated oven for 25-30 minutes, until tender and golden brown.

Cucumber and Tomato Salad

Ingredients:

- 2 thinly sliced cucumbers

- 1 cup cherry tomatoes (halved)

- 1/4 cup thinly sliced red onion.

- Ingredients:

- 2 tablespoons chopped fresh dill,

- 2 tablespoons olive oil, and

- 1 tablespoon red wine vinegar.

- Add salt and pepper to taste.

Instructions:

1. In a large mixing bowl, combine sliced cucumbers, halved cherry tomatoes, sliced red onion, and fresh dill.
2. Dress with olive oil and red wine vinegar.
3. Season with salt and pepper.
4. Before serving, toss the ingredients until thoroughly combined.

Sautéed Spinach with Garlic

Ingredients:

- 4 cups baby spinach and

- 2 minced garlic cloves.

- One tablespoon of olive oil.

- Season with salt and pepper to taste.

Instructions:

1. Heat the olive oil in a large skillet over medium heat.
2. Add the minced garlic and cook for about 1 minute, until fragrant.
3. Cook the baby spinach in the skillet until wilted, about 2-3 minutes.
4. Sprinkle with salt and pepper before serving.

Greek Salad

Ingredients:

- 2 cups chopped romaine lettuce,
- 1 diced cucumber, and
- 1 cup halved cherry tomatoes.
- 1/4 cup thinly sliced red onion.
- 1/4 cup Kalamata olives
- Add 1/4 cup crumbled feta cheese,
- 2 tablespoons chopped fresh parsley,
- 2 tablespoons olive oil, and
- 1 tablespoon red wine vinegar.

- Add salt and pepper to taste.

Instructions:

1. In a large mixing bowl, combine the chopped romaine lettuce, diced cucumber, halved cherry tomatoes, sliced red onion, Kalamata olives, crumbled feta cheese, and chopped fresh parsley.
2. Dress with olive oil and red wine vinegar.
3. Season with salt and pepper.
4. Before serving, toss the ingredients until thoroughly combined.

Roasted Brussels sprouts with Balsamic Glaze

Ingredients:

- 2 cups of halved Brussels sprouts
- 1 tablespoon olive oil
- Season with salt and pepper to taste.

- Add 2 tablespoons of balsamic glaze.

Instructions:

1. Preheat your oven to 400°F (200°C).
2. Toss the halved Brussels sprouts with olive oil, salt, and pepper until well coated.
3. Arrange the Brussels sprouts in a single layer on a baking sheet.
4. Roast in a preheated oven for 20-25 minutes, until tender and caramelized.
5. Drizzle with balsamic glaze before serving.

Tagbouleh Salad

Ingredients:

- 1 cup cooked bulgur wheat,
- 1 diced cucumber, and
- 1 cup halved cherry tomatoes.
- 1/4 cup finely chopped red onion.
- Add 1/4 cup chopped fresh parsley and 2 tablespoons chopped fresh mint.

- Two tablespoons of olive oil.

- Juice from 1 lemon

- Season with salt and pepper to taste.

Instructions:

- In a large mixing bowl, combine cooked bulgur wheat, diced cucumber, halved cherry tomatoes, finely chopped red onion, chopped fresh parsley, and fresh mint.

- Drizzle with olive oil and lemon juice.

- Season with salt and pepper.

- Before serving, toss the ingredients until thoroughly combined.

Roasted Cauliflower with Turmeric

Ingredients:

- 1 head cauliflower,

- cut into florets

- 2 tablespoons olive oil

- 1 teaspoon ground turmeric

- 1/2 teaspoon ground cumin.
- Season with salt and pepper to taste.

Instructions:

1. Pre-heat the oven to 425°F (220°C).
2. Toss cauliflower florets with olive oil, ground turmeric, ground cumin, salt, and pepper until well combined.
3. Arrange the cauliflower in a single layer on a baking sheet.
4. Roast in a preheated oven for 25-30 minutes, until tender and golden brown.

Mixed bean salad

Ingredients:

1. 1 can (15 ounces) mixed beans, drained and rinsed (e.g. kidney beans, black beans, chickpeas).
2. Add 1/2 cup diced bell pepper,

3. 1/4 cup diced red onion, and 2 tablespoons chopped fresh cilantro.

4. Add 2 tablespoons olive oil and

5. 1 tablespoon red wine vinegar.

6. Season with salt and pepper to taste.

Instructions:

1. In a large bowl, combine the mixed beans, diced bell pepper, diced red onion, and chopped fresh cilantro.

2. Mixed Bean Salad (continued)

3. Instructions (continued):

4. In a small bowl, combine the olive oil, red wine vinegar, salt, and pepper.

5. Drizzle the dressing over the bean mix.

6. Toss until thoroughly combined.

7. Marinate the salad in the refrigerator for at least 30 minutes before serving to allow the flavors to combine.

Grilled Veggie Platter

Ingredients:

- 1 sliced zucchini,
- 1 sliced yellow squash, and
- 1 sliced eggplant.
- Quarter one red and one yellow bell pepper.
- One tablespoon of olive oil.
- Add salt and pepper to taste. - Drizzle with balsamic glaze (optional).

Instructions:

1. Preheat the grill to medium-high.
2. Drizzle olive oil over sliced vegetables and season with salt and pepper.
3. Grill the vegetables for 3-5 minutes on each side, or until tender and charred.
4. Arrange the grilled vegetables on a platter.
5. If desired, drizzle with balsamic glaze just before serving.

Cauliflower rice pilaf

Ingredients:

- 1 head of cauliflower,
- grated into rice-like texture.
- Add 2 tablespoons olive oil,
- 1/4 cup diced onion, and 1/4 cup diced carrots.
- 1/4 cup frozen peas (thawed)
- 2 garlic cloves, minced
- 1/4 cup chopped fresh parsley.
- Season with salt and pepper to taste.

Instructions:

1. Heat the olive oil in a large skillet over medium heat.
2. Cook the diced onion and carrots in the skillet until they soften.
3. Stir in the minced garlic and cook for an additional minute.

4. Add the grated cauliflower to the skillet and cook until tender, about 5-7 minutes.

5. Stir in the frozen peas and chopped fresh parsley.

6. Sprinkle with salt and pepper before serving.

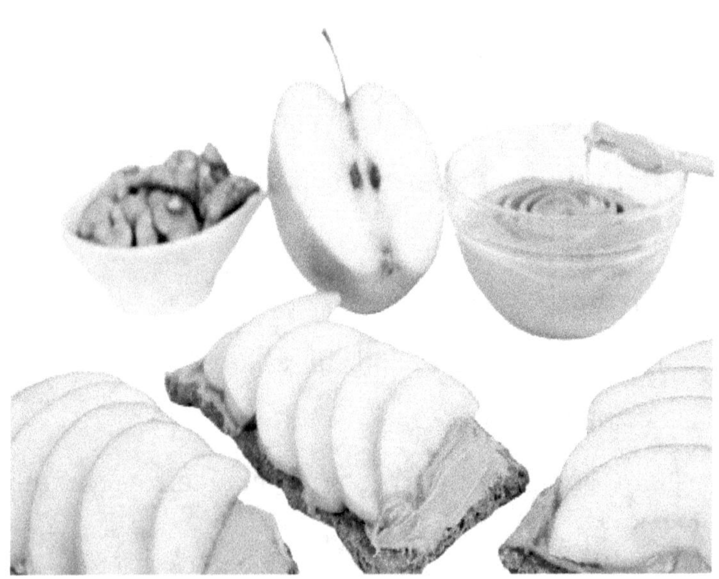

Chapter 6: Desserts

Berry Parfait

Ingredients:

- 1 cup mixed berries (strawberries, blueberries, raspberries) and
- 1 cup Greek yogurt.
- 1 tablespoon honey, 1/4 cup granola.

Instructions:

1. In serving glasses, arrange the mixed berries, Greek yogurt, and honey.
2. Repeat the layers until the glasses are full.
3. Top with granola.
4. Serve chilled.

Baked apples with cinnamon

Ingredients:

- 2 cored apples

- 2 tablespoons of chopped walnuts

- Add 1 tablespoon honey and

- 1/2 teaspoon ground cinnamon.

Instructions:

1. Preheat your oven to 375°F (190°C).

2. Place the cored apples on a baking dish.

3. In a bowl, combine the chopped walnuts, honey, and ground cinnamon.

4. Stuff the mixture into the cored apples.

5. Bake for 20–25 minutes, or until apples are tender.

6. Serve warm.

Dark chocolate-covered strawberries

Ingredients:

- 8 strawberries (rinsed and dried)

- 2 ounces chopped dark chocolate

Instructions:

1. In a microwave-safe bowl, melt dark chocolate at 30-second intervals while stirring until smooth.

2. Dip each strawberry in melted chocolate, coating halfway.

3. Place on a parchment-lined baking sheet.

4. Chill in the refrigerator until the chocolate has set.

5. Serve chilled.

Frozen Yogurt Bark

Ingredients:

- 2 cups of Greek yogurt.
- 1 tablespoon honey, 1/4 cup mixed berries (blueberries, raspberries), and 1/4 cup granola.

Instructions:

1. In a bowl, combine Greek yogurt and honey.

2. Line a baking sheet with parchment paper.

3. Spread the yogurt mixture evenly on the parchment paper.

4. Top the yogurt with mixed berries and granola.

5. Freeze for 2–3 hours, or until firm.

6. Divide into pieces and serve cold.

Chia Seed Pudding

Ingredients:

- 1/4 cup chia seeds
- 1 cup unsweetened almond milk
- 1 tablespoon honey
- 1/2 teaspoon vanilla extract
- Optional topping with fresh fruit.

Instructions:

1. In a bowl, combine the chia seeds, almond milk, honey, and vanilla extract.

2. Cover and refrigerate for at least 2 hours, or overnight, to thicken.

3. Give it a good stir before serving.

4. Garnish with fresh fruit if desired.

Banana Oat Cookies

Ingredients:

- 2 ripe bananas (mashed)
- One cup rolled oats.
- 1/4 cup chopped nuts (walnuts or almonds)
- 1/4 cup of dark chocolate chips (optional).

Instructions:

1. Preheat the oven to 350°F/175°C.

2. In a bowl, combine the mashed bananas, rolled oats, chopped nuts, and dark chocolate chips (if using).

3. Spoon spoonfuls of the mixture onto a parchment-lined baking sheet.

4. Flatten using a fork.

5. Bake for 12–15 minutes, or until golden brown.

6. Let cool before serving.

Fruit Salad With Mint Honey Dressing

Ingredients:

- 2 cups mixed fruit (pineapple, grapes, kiwi, and orange segments).
- 2 tablespoons of fresh mint leaves, chopped
- One tablespoon of honey.

Instructions:

1. In a mixing bowl, combine the fruit and chopped mint leaves.
2. Drizzle honey on the fruit salad.
3. Gently toss until evenly coated.
4. Serve chilled.

Coconut-Mango Rice Pudding

Ingredients :

- 1/2 cup cooked brown rice and

- 1/2 cup coconut milk.

- Add 1/4 cup diced mango,

- 1 tablespoon shredded coconut, and

- 1 tablespoon honey.

Instructions:

1. In a saucepan, combine the cooked brown rice and coconut milk.

2. Cook over medium heat until thoroughly heated.

3. Mix in the diced mango, shredded coconut, and honey.

4. Cook for an additional 2-3 minutes, or until the mixture has thickened.

5. Serve either warm or chilled.

Greek Yogurt Popsicles

Ingredients:

- 1 cup Greek yogurt

- 1/4 cup mixed berries (blueberries and strawberries)
- 1 tablespoon honey

Instructions:

1. In a bowl, combine the Greek yogurt, mixed berries, and honey.
2. Pour the mixture into the popsicle molds.
3. Insert the popsicle sticks.
4. Freeze for 4-6 hours, or until solid.

Almond Date Bites

Ingredients:

- One cup pitted dates.
- One cup almonds.
- Two tablespoons of unsweetened cocoa powder.
- 1 teaspoon vanilla extract - 1/4 cup shredded coconut (optional for coating).

Instructions:

1. In a food processor, mix together pitted dates, almonds, cocoa powder, and vanilla extract.

2. Pulse the ingredients until they form a sticky dough.

3. Roll the dough into small balls.

4. Optionally, coat each ball with shredded coconut.

5. Transfer the almond date bites to an airtight container and chill for at least 30 minutes before serving.

Apple Cinnamon Oatmeal Cookie

Ingredients:

- 1 cup rolled oats, 1/2 cup unsweetened applesauce, and 1/4 cup almond butter.

- 1/4 cup chopped dried apples.

- Add 2 tablespoons of honey and 1 teaspoon of ground cinnamon.

- 1/2 teaspoon of vanilla extract.

Instructions:

1. Preheat the oven to 350°F/175°C and line a baking sheet with parchment paper.

2. In a mixing bowl, combine the rolled oats, unsweetened applesauce, almond butter, chopped dried apples, honey, ground cinnamon, and vanilla extract.

3. Mix until thoroughly combined.

4. Drop spoonfuls of the dough onto the prepared baking sheet, flattening each one slightly with the back of a spoon.

5. Bake for 12–15 minutes, or until golden brown.

6. Let the cookies cool on the baking sheet for 5 minutes before transferring to a wire rack to finish cooling.

7. Enjoy these nutritious and tasty treats!

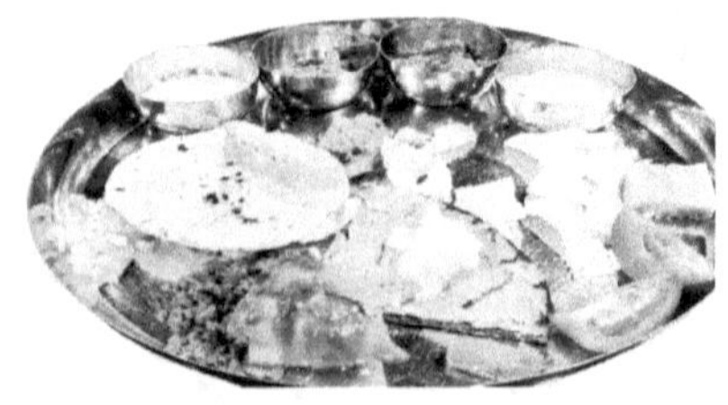

Chapter 7: Appetizers and Snacks

avocado toast

Ingredients:

- One ripe avocado.
- 2 slices of whole grain bread and 1 teaspoon lemon juice.
- Season with salt and pepper to taste.

Instructions:

1. Toast the whole-grain bread slices until golden brown.
2. Mash the ripe avocados with lemon juice, salt, and pepper.
3. Spread the mashed avocado mixture evenly across the toasted bread slices.
4. Serve immediately.

Greek Yogurt Dip and Fresh Vegetables

Ingredients:

- 1 cup Greek yogurt
- 1 clove garlic, minced
- One tablespoon of lemon juice.
- 1 tablespoon chopped fresh dill
- Fresh vegetables (carrots, cucumber, bell peppers) for dipping

Instructions:

- In a bowl, combine Greek yogurt, garlic, lemon juice, and fresh dill.
- Serve the Greek yogurt dip alongside various fresh vegetables for dipping.

Smoked Salmon Cucumber Bite

Ingredients:

- English cucumber,
- cut into rounds.

- Four ounces of smoked salmon

- Two tablespoons of cream cheese.

- Fresh dill as garnish

Instructions:

1. Spread a small amount of cream cheese onto each cucumber round.

2. Finish with a piece of smoked salmon.

3. Sprinkle with fresh dill before serving.

Hummus-stuffed mini bell peppers

Ingredients:

- 12 mini bell peppers.

- 1/2 cup hummus

- Fresh parsley for garnish

instructions:

1. Cut off the tops of the mini bell peppers and remove the seeds.

2. Fill each pepper with hummus.

3. Prior to serving, garnish with fresh parsley.

caprese skewers

Ingredients:

- cherry tomatoes and fresh mozzarella balls.
- Fresh basil leaves.
- balsamic glaze, toothpicks, and

instructions.

1. Thread a cherry tomato, a mozzarella ball, and a fresh basil leaf on each toothpick.
2. Place the skewers on a serving platter.
3. Drizzle with balsamic glaze before serving.

Edamame with Sea Salt

Ingredients:

- 1 cup frozen edamame (thawed)
- Add sea salt to taste. - Instructions:
- Heat a pot of water to a boil.

- Cook the thawed edamame for 3-5 minutes.
- Drain the edamame and season with sea salt before serving.

Quinoa-stuffed mushrooms

Ingredients:

- 12 large mushrooms with stems removed
- 1 cup cooked quinoa
- 1/4 cup diced red bell pepper
- 1/4 cup diced onion
- 1 minced clove of garlic
- 1 tablespoon olive oil
- 2 tablespoons grated Parmesan cheese
- Salt and pepper to taste

Instructions:

1. Preheat the oven to 375°F (190°C), then lightly grease a baking sheet.
2. In a skillet, heat the olive oil over medium heat.

3. Cook the diced onion and red bell pepper in the skillet until softened.

4. Add the minced garlic and cook for another minute.

5. Stir in the cooked quinoa, grated Parmesan cheese, salt, and pepper.

6. Transfer the quinoa mixture to the mushroom caps.

7. Transfer the stuffed mushrooms to the prepared baking sheet and bake for 15-20 minutes, or until tender.

8. Serve warm.

Baked Kale Chips

Ingredients:

- 1 bunch kale (stems removed and torn into bite-sized pieces).
- 1 tablespoon olive oil
- Salt and pepper to taste - Recipe

instructions:

1. Preheat the oven to 275°F/135°C and line a baking sheet with parchment paper.

2. In a large mixing bowl, toss kale with olive oil, salt, and pepper until evenly coated.

3. Arrange the kale in a single layer on the prepared baking sheet.

4. Bake for 20 to 25 minutes, or until the kale is crispy.

5. Let cool before serving.

Bruschetta with tomatoes and basil

Ingredients:

- 4 slices whole grain baguette,
- 2 diced ripe tomatoes, and
- 2 minced garlic cloves.
- 2 tablespoons chopped fresh basil,
- 1 tablespoon balsamic vinegar.
- Season with salt and pepper to taste.

Instructions:

1. Toast the slices of whole grain baguette until they are lightly golden.
2. In a mixing bowl, combine diced tomatoes, garlic, chopped fresh basil, balsamic vinegar, salt, and pepper.
3. Spoon the tomato mixture over the toasted baguette slices.
4. Serve immediately.

Stuffed celery with almond butter

Ingredients:

- 4 celery stalks (cut into 3-inch pieces)
- 1/4 cup almond butter
- 2 tablespoons raisins.

Instructions:

1. Apply almond butter to the hollow part of each celery stalk.
2. Top with raisins.

3. Serve chilled.

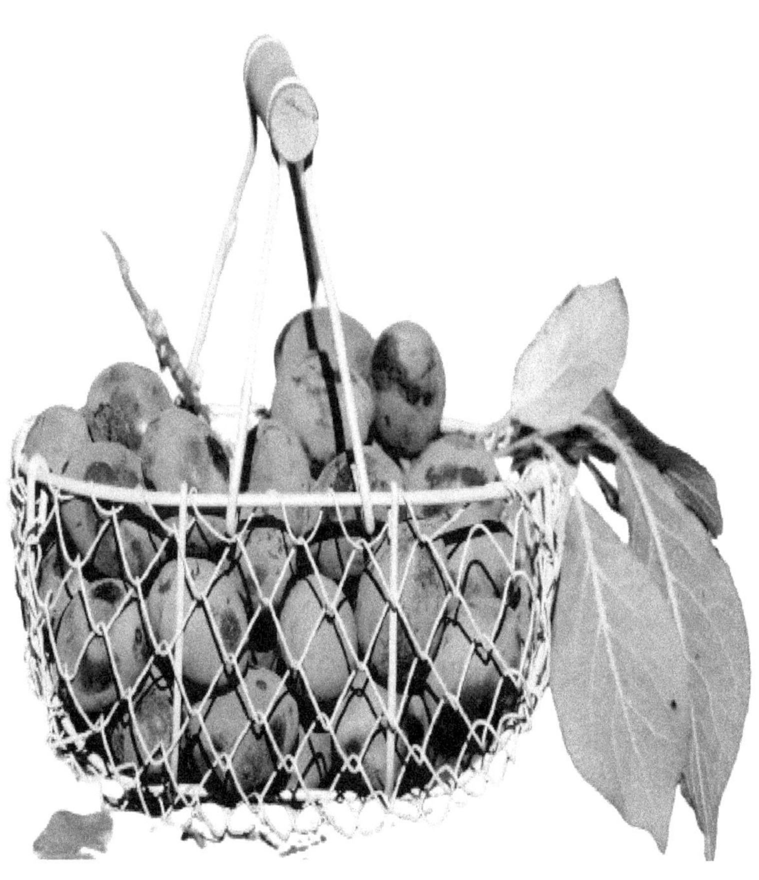

Chapter 7: Beverages

Green Smoothie

Ingredients:

- 1 cup spinach
- 1/2 cup kale
- One-half banana
- 1/2 cup pineapple chunks
- Half cup unsweetened almond milk
- One tablespoon of chia seeds (optional)

Instructions:

- Combine all of the ingredients in a blender.
- Blend until smooth and creamy.
- Serve immediately.

Berry Blast Smoothie

Ingredients:

- 1/2 cup mixed berries (strawberries, blueberries, and raspberries).

- One-half banana

- Half cup Greek yogurt

- Half cup unsweetened almond milk

- One tablespoon of honey (optional).

Instructions:

- Combine all ingredients in a blender.

- Blend until smooth.

- Taste and add honey if desired.

- Serve cold.

Turmeric Golden Milk

Ingredients:

- 1 cup unsweetened almond milk,

- 1/2 teaspoon ground turmeric, and

- 1/4 teaspoon ground cinnamon.

- 1/4 teaspoon ground ginger.

- One teaspoon of honey (optional)

Instructions:

1. Cook almond milk in a small saucepan over medium heat until warm but not boiling.

2. Mix in the ground turmeric, cinnamon, and ginger.

3. If desired, add honey and stir until dissolved.

4. Transfer to a mug and serve hot.

Iced Green Tea

Ingredients:

- Two green tea bags.

- 2 cups of water - Ice cubes.

- Lemon slices as garnish (optional)

Instructions:

1. Bring water to a boil in a saucepan.

2. Remove from heat and add the green tea bags.

3. Steep for 3 to 5 minutes.

4. Remove the teabags and allow the tea to cool to room temperature.

5. Pour the tea into glasses containing ice cubes.

6. Garnish with lemon slices if desired.

7. Serve chilled.

Coconut Water Smoothie

Ingredients:

- 1 cup coconut water,
- 1/2 cup frozen mango chunks.
- 1/2 cup frozen pineapple cubes
- One-half banana

Instructions:

1. Combine all of the ingredients in a blender.

2. Blend until smooth.

3. Transfer to a glass and serve cold.

Lemon Ginger Detox Water

Ingredients:

- 4 cups water,
- 1 sliced lemon,
- 1 thinly sliced ginger,
- and fresh mint leaves.

Instructions:

1. In a pitcher, combine water, lemon and ginger slices, and fresh mint leaves.
2. Refrigerate for at least an hour to allow the flavors to blend.
3. Serve chilled with ice.

Cucumber Mint-Infused Water

Ingredients:

- 4 cups of water
- 1/2 sliced cucumber.

Instructions:

1. In a pitcher, mix together water, cucumber slices, and fresh mint leaves.
2. Refrigerate for at least an hour to allow the flavors to blend.
3. Serve chilled with ice.

Homemade Lemonade

Ingredients:

- 4 cups water
- 1/2 cup freshly squeezed lemon juice.
- 1/4 cup honey
- Lemon slices as garnish (optional)

Instructions:

1. In a pitcher, mix together water, fresh lemon juice, and honey.
2. Stir until the honey has dissolved.
3. Refrigerate for at least an hour to chill.

4. Serve over ice, garnished with lemon slices if desired.

Berry-Hibiscus Iced Tea

Ingredients:

- Two hibiscus tea bags.
- Add 2 cups boiling water,
- 1/2 cup mixed berries (strawberries, raspberries, blueberries), and ice cubes.

Instructions:

1. Place the hibiscus tea bags in a heatproof pitcher.
2. Pour boiling water over the tea bags, then steep for 5-7 minutes.
3. Remove the tea bags and cool the tea to room temperature.
4. Add the mixed berries to the pitcher.
5. Chill for at least an hour to allow the flavors to infuse.

6. Serve over ice.

Pineapple Coconut Water

Ingredients:

- 2 cups coconut water
- 1 cup of pineapple juice
- 1/2 cup sparkling water.
- Pineapple slices as garnish (optional)

Instructions:

1. In a pitcher, mix the coconut water and pineapple juice.
2. Stir in the sparkling water.
3. Refrigerate for at least an hour to chill.
4. If desired, serve over ice with pineapple slices as garnish.

Chapter 8: 14-Day Meal for the seniors mind diet

Day 1:

Breakfast: Berry oatmeal with walnuts.

Lunch: Mediterranean Chickpea Salad.

Dinner: Baked salmon with roasted vegetables.

Day 2:

Breakfast: Spinach and Feta Omelet.

Lunch: Quinoa-stuffed bell peppers.

Dinner: Lemon Herb Chicken and Steamed Broccoli

Day 3:

Breakfast: Greek Yogurt Parfait with Mixed Berries.

Lunch: Lentil Soup and Whole Grain Bread

Dinner: Grilled Turkey Burgers and Sweet Potato Fries.

Day 4:

Breakfast: Avocado toast with poached eggs.

Lunch: Tuna salad. Wrap with a whole grain tortilla.

Dinner: Vegetable stir-fry with brown rice.

Day 5:

Breakfast: Banana Almond Smoothie.

Lunch: Caprese salad with balsamic glaze.

Dinner: Herb-roasted pork tenderloin with quinoa pilaf.

Day 6:

Breakfast: Whole grain pancakes with fresh fruit.

Lunch: chicken Caesar salad.

Dinner: Ratatouille and Grilled Chicken Breast

Day 7:

Breakfast: Chia Seed Pudding with Mango Slices.

Lunch: Greek lentil salad.

Dinner: Baked cod with asparagus and lemon butter sauce.

Day 8:

Breakfast: Spinach and Mushroom Frittata.

Lunch: Hummus and Veggie Wrap; *Dinner:* Turkey Meatballs with Zucchini Noodles.

Day 9:

Breakfast: Blueberry Walnut Overnight Oatmeal.

Lunch: Quinoa and black bean salad.

Dinner: Baked Halibut with Roasted Brussels sprouts.

Day 10:

Breakfast: Green smoothie bowl with granola.

Lunch: Mediterranean Veggie Wrap *Dinner:* Lemon Garlic Shrimp and Cauliflower Rice

Day 11:

Breakfast: Yogurt Berry Bowl with Almond Butter.

Lunch: Spinach and strawberry salad with grilled chicken

Dinner: Beef and Vegetable Kabobs with Herbal Quinoa

Day 12:

Breakfast: Veggie Egg Muffins.

Lunch: Chickpea and Spinach Stuffed Sweet Potatoes.

Dinner: Salmon Burgers and Cucumber Salad

Day 13:

Breakfast: Peanut Butter Banana Toast.

Lunch: Greek orzo salad.

Dinner: Balsamic-glazed chicken with roasted vegetables.

Day 14:

we had Apple Cinnamon Baked Oatmeal for breakfast and a Mediterranean Hummus Plate with Whole Wheat Pita for lunch.

Dinner: Spaghetti squash primavera with grilled shrimp.

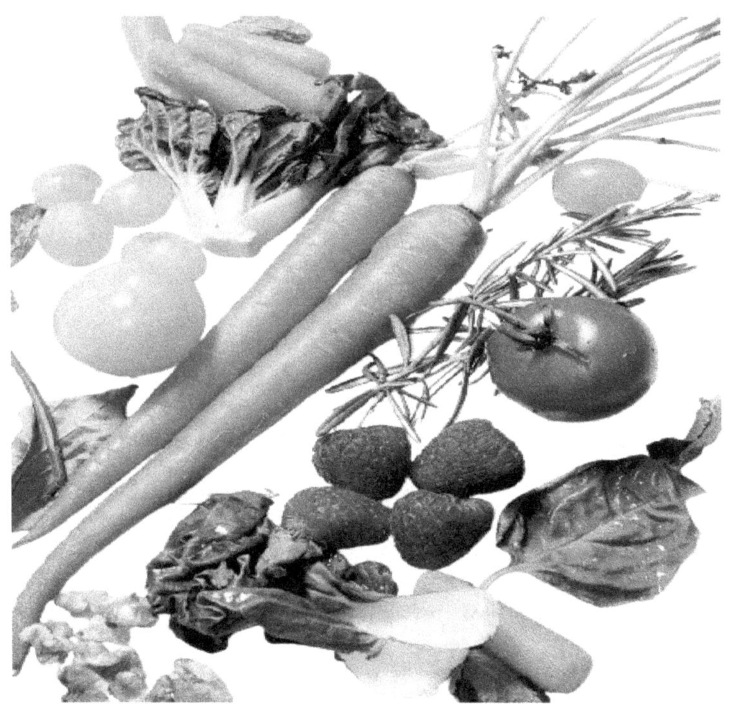

Conclusion

To summarize, the Mind Diet Cookbook for Seniors Over 60 is an invaluable resource for promoting brain health, improving cognitive function, and nourishing the body with delicious and nutrient-dense meals. Seniors can improve their well-being and vitality by understanding the Mind Diet principles. Seniors can enjoy a variety of meals while reaping the benefits of this brain-boosting diet, thanks to an array of appetizing recipes tailored specifically to their dietary needs and preferences.

Additional resources

1. *Mind Diet:* A Comprehensive Guide - This comprehensive guide provides detailed information about the Mind Diet, including its origins, scientific research, and practical implementation tips. It offers useful insights into the dietary principles and

lifestyle factors that influence cognitive health and longevity.

2. *Mindful Eating for Seniors:* A Practical Guide. This book focuses on mindful eating, which builds on the Mind Diet's principles by encouraging seniors to become more aware of their food choices and eating habits. It contains mindfulness exercises, meal planning strategies, and mindful eating practices designed specifically for seniors.

3. *Brain Health and Aging:* A Guide for Seniors. This guide, written by geriatric medicine and neuroscience experts, provides valuable information on how to keep your brain healthy as you get older. It discusses cognitive exercises, lifestyle modifications, and dietary recommendations, as well as the Mind Diet principles.

4. Cooking for One or Two Cookbook: Simple, Healthy Recipes for Seniors - This cookbook is ideal for seniors living alone or with a partner because it contains simple and nutritious recipes that are easy to prepare and perfectly portioned for small households. It offers a variety of meal options, such as breakfasts, lunches, dinners, and snacks, all tailored to the dietary needs of seniors.

5. Mindful Living: A Daily Journal for Seniors – This guided journal helps seniors practice mindfulness and self-reflection in their daily lives. With prompts, exercises, and inspirational quotes, it encourages seniors to engage in mindful practices that promote overall well-being, such as mindful eating as part of the Mind Diet approach.